THE MINDSET OF THE WINNING DIET

How to be the

Best Version of Yourself

ADAM CLARK

or directions contained within is the solitary and utter responsibility of the recipient reader. Under no circumstances will any legal responsibility or blame be held against the publisher for any reparation, damages, or monetary loss due to the information herein, either directly or indirectly.

Respective authors own all copyrights not held by the publisher.

The information herein is offered for informational purposes solely, and is universal as so. The presentation of the information is without contract or any type of guarantee assurance.

The trademarks that are used are without any consent, and the publication of the trademark is without permission or backing by the trademark owner. All trademarks and brands within this book are for clarifying purposes only and are the owned by the owners themselves, not affiliated with this document.

Table of Content

INTRODUCTION

In many people around the world, excess weight or obesity is a chronic partner. The truth is that most people simply do not know which weight loss diets are the most successful and end up getting sick rather than losing weight. Many others do not have independent power and can remain in an effective weight loss system before long. These are all issues arising from incompetence and insufficient weight loss knowledge.

Because of today's limitless weight loss choices, the choice of the best weight loss plan or diet for you is challenging. The decision is more perplexing as there are so many substitutes such as food, workouts and weight loss supplements and other choices. It is therefore important that consumers choose a weight loss program that lets them lose weight, but that helps them stay well. To order to achieve an optimal weight loss plan, both safety and fitness must be combined.

Any weight loss option that causes the body to fail or any health problems should be avoided. The mixture of healthy diets and workouts is one of the easiest ways to lose weight and maintain good health.

Note, it is not possible for you to reach a healthy weight loss by incorporating these choices. You should try and eat well to stop hunger or vomiting, as this only adds to further health issues for you.

Various options and diets are available today for rapid weight loss. Such diets favor the consumer in a short time of drastic quick weight loss, which would be enticing to most.

Some fast weight loss diets say that in a matter of days they will help you lose weight. Nonetheless, it is not good enough for any diet because even such fast diets for weight loss come at an expense. This quality may not always be economical, but also safe and healthy. Choose foods that can be fried or eaten raw can be used for certain diets only to eat chosen fruit or vegetables. The process of cooking also has to be tested if you intend to prepare these fruits and vegetables.

The best way to eat regular yet healthy meals is for the body's metabolic rate to be high. Hunger often raises fat deposits in the body, allowing you to become fatter in the longer term. Fat and starch should be taken at least 6 times to lose weight.

A realistic target must be considered in order to lose weight effectively. Many individuals who start on a diet plan either fail to formulate the right strategy or seek to meet ambitious weight loss expectations to achieve their goals. The effectiveness of any weight loss plan will be measured according to the time and commitment. When your success improves and the pounds begin to drop, you feel stronger and stronger, and eventually your wellbeing will feel better. May anger not preclude you from fulfilling "the bulge's challenge" your goals.

Morning Habits That Help You Lose Weight

Regardless of your weight loss goals, weight loss may sometimes feel impossible. Your present diet and lifestyle should not, though, be completely overhauled for a few pounds.

In reality it can help you lose weight and hold it off with a few small changes to your morning routine. Here are the simple morning ways to suit your diet and help you lose weight.

1. Eat a High-Protein Breakfast

There is a reason that breakfast is considered the most important meal of the day. Eat High-Protein Breakfast. You will set the course for the whole day for what you eat for breakfast. This decides whether you will feel satisfied until lunch, or whether you will go to the store before your mid-morning snack.

A high protein breakfast can help lower your cravings and help you to lose your weight. For one test, eating a high protein breakfast for 20 adolescent girls decreased the afternoon cravings better than having a regular protein breakfast. The minor study has found, compared to a normal protein breakfast that eating a high protein breakfast has decreased fat gain and a reduced daily consumption and appetite.

The "hunger hormone," which is responsible for increasing appetite, can also promote weight loss with reduced ghrelin levels. Yes, a study conducted in 15 men found that a high protein breakfast more efficiently reduces ghrelin secretion than a low-carb breakfast. Include protein sources, such as bacon, Greek yogurt, cottage cheese, and chia seeds to help get your day off to a good start.

2. Drink plenty of water

The easiest way to improve weight loss is to begin the morning with a glass or two of tea. For at least 60 minutes, water will help to increase the energy consumption or the number of calories that your body burns.

For one small study, a 30% boost for metabolism was accomplished by consuming 16,9 fluid ounces (500 ml) of water on average. Another research has shown that an estimated 4.4 pounds (2 kg) over a one year span has been wasted among overweight women or men who raised their water consumption to about 34 ounces (one liter) per day, without any further adjustments in diet or exercise.

In fact, certain people may experience a decrease in appetite and consumption of food.

A survey of 24 older adults found a 13% decrease in the amount of calories eaten in the breakfast by consuming 16.9 fluid onces (500 ml) of tea. In fact, most of the studies showed that drinking water per day for 34–68 ounces (1–2 liters) would assist in the loss of weight. It is a great way to boost weight loss with minimum effort to start the morning with water and remain well moistured throughout the day.

3. Weighing yourself

Every morning can be a successful way of increasing your confidence and self-control. Weigh yourself several studies have linked to a higher weight loss every day.

A research of 47 people showed, for example, that those who weighed each other more than those who weighed themselves less often lost about 13 pounds (6 kg) a day in six months. Another research report suggested that people with a daily weigh of 9.7 pounds (4.4 kg) were losing for two years on average, while those with a weekly weight gained 4.6 kilograms (2.1 kg).

You can also promote healthy activities and routines that can facilitate weight loss each morning. Frequently self-weighing with increased control has been correlated in a large study. In fact, people who stopped being measured more often show higher calorie intake and diminished self-discipline.

Weigh yourself right as you wake up to the best performance. Do this before you eat or drink anything after use of the toilet. However, note that your weight will fluctuate every day and depend on several factors.

Concentrate on the large scene and try general impulses to lose weight, rather than focusing on small changes daily.

4. Get some Sun

Get some sun to continue your weight loss by opening your curtains to encourage some sunshine or to leave for a few extra minutes every day. One small study showed that even low light levels would affect weight at certain times of the day.

In fact, researchers found that ultra-violet radiation exposure helped reduce weight gain in mice, which ate a high-fat diet. The best way to meet the vitamin D needs is by exposure to sunlight. Several studies have found that it can improve weight loss and reduce weight gain by fulfilling the vitamin D requirements.

218 overweight and obese women received either one year in one research vitamin D supplements or one year in placebo. At the conclusion of the research, those with insufficient levels of blood vitamin D lost 7 pounds (3.2 kg), on average, rather than those with an inappropriate level of vitamin D.

Another study was conducted by 4,659 older women over 4 years. Higher vitamin D levels were associated with reduced weight gain. Based on your type of skin, season and place, the amount of sunlight you need can vary. Nonetheless, preparing for 10–15 minutes every morning in sunshine or sitting outdoors can have a positive impact on weight loss.

5. Practice Mindfulness

Mindfulness is a practice that involves fully focusing on the present moment and bringing awareness to your thoughts and feelings. The practice has been shown to enhance weight loss and promote healthy eating habits.

The review of 19 studies showed, for example, that knowledge based approaches improved weight loss and reduced eating behavior associated with obesity.

The study found that conscientiousness preparation resulted in a significant weight loss in 68% of the studied trials. It's quick to cultivate consciousness. To get going, try sitting comfortably in quiet rooms and engaging the senses for five minutes every morning.

6. Squeeze in some workout

The first thing in the morning will help increase the loss of weight. One research of fifty women with overweight measured at different times of the day the impact of aerobic activity.

Although there was no distinction between those who trained in the morning and the afternoon in specific foods, exercising in the morning was associated with greater satiety. Exercise in the morning will help to maintain blood sugar levels stable all day long. Low blood sugar, like intense appetite, can contribute to many negative symptoms. A study conducted in 35 individuals with type 1 diabetes found a greater blood sugar control in the morning.

7. Packaging your lunch

You should prepare and pack your lunch in advance by making healthier food choices and increasing the loss of weight. A large study of 40,554 participants showed a better quality of eating, improved nutrition and reduced risk of obesity. food preparation has been related.

The study showed that intake of prepared foods was more regular due to better health and a lower risk of excess body fat. However, 28 percent less likely to be overweighted for those who eaten home-cooked meals at least five days a week than those who ate homemade meals just three times or less a week.

Taking a couple hours a night to schedule your meals and cook them in order to grab your lunch and leave in the morning.

8. Sleep Longer

If you go to bed a little early or set an alarm clock for a little extra sleep, weight loss can improve. Several studies have found a stronger tolerance for sleep deprivation.

A small study showed that sleep constraints increased malnutrition and hunger, in particular for high-carbon, high-calorie foods. Sleep loss is also related to a rise in calorie consumption.

12 subjects ate a total of 559 more calories in one study after only four hours of sleep, compared to 8 hours.

A healthy sleep routine is a critical component of loss of weight and good food and exercise. Achieve at least 8 hours of sleep per night to optimize your performance. Such experiments, however, have concentrated on highly specific populations and have a correlation instead of a source. Further research is needed on the impact of morning workouts in the general public.

9. Change your shuttle to work

While commuting may not be one of the most comfortable ways of getting to work. Research indicates that walking, cycling or public transport can be associated with lower body weight and a lower risk of weight gain.

A four-year survey tracked 822 people and found that travelers traveling by car tend to gain more weight than drivers.

Furthermore, a survey of 15,777 people showed that the body density and body fat level were considerably lower relative to the use of private transport than public transport or alternative means of transportation, such as walking or biking. It can be an easy way to increase weight loss just a few days per week if you change your path.

10. Track your diet

The keeping of a food journal to track what you're consuming will help increase weight loss and be responsible. One research study recorded weight loss in 123 participants for a year and observed a greater weight loss in the completion of a food journal.

The study showed that participants with a tracking system to automatically control their diet and exercise were losing weight more than participants without the tracking system on a regular basis.

Likewise, the frequent and regular use of a self-monitoring device has been shown by a survey of 220 obese women to improve their weight management in the long term. Attempt to remember, beginning with your first meal of the day, with an app, or even only a pen and paper.

Ways to Shift Your Mindset for Better Weight Loss

Each good diet and plan for weight loss has its advantages and disadvantages, but, for everyone to succeed, you have to think correctly.

"The greatest factor in weight loss is to change your perspective on how to lose weight," researchers said: Most people are trying to lose weight in a worst imaginable state of mind: they want to "correct" it themselves. "We don't want to change our weight from the outside by having a right inner determination yet purpose."

You leap on diets and exercise plans out of self-deprecation and grab your "disorderly" points all the while, mark yourself "fat" and feel absolutely less like that. We become obsessed with results, rely on quick solutions and lose sight of sustainability and safety.

"This type of thinking could be detrimental, " these people rely on negative thoughts rather than concentrating on what may be positive about losing weight–such as improved health, a longer life, more enjoyment at everyday activities and avoiding diabetes and heart disease.

Essentially, the negative attitude triggers a collapse. "Well, changing the mindset toward the weight loss doesn't only involve getting lustful; it's about performance. Fortunately, the mind is a flexible thing.

Here are the expert-approved tips to change your mindset and make your weight-loss approach healthier, happier and way more effective:

1. Change Your Goals

Losing weight might be a result, but it shouldn't be the goal. Rather, your goals should small, sustainable things over which you have full control, Did you eat five servings of fruits and veggies today? There's one goal met. What about eight hours of sleep; did you get them in? If so, you can check another goal off of your list.

2. Gravitate to Positivity

"Surround yourself with positive people," Doing so provides you an encouraging, emotionally healthy environment in which to invest in yourself. "Don't be afraid to ask for help or support.

3. Rethink Rewards and Punishments

"Since making healthy decisions is a way of self-care, diet does not mean a recompense and exercise is no penalty. Rethink bonuses and fines." Both of them help you to take care of your body and look the best. You're both worth it.

4. Take a Breath

Calm down and simply concentrate on the breathing process, take a few minutes to begin your exercise or even early in the day, will help set your objectives, link up with your body and reduce the body's pressure, researchers say. Take a breath. Lied down with your legs spread and put your stomach with a hand and shoulders with one hand. Respire in the nose for four seconds, keep for two and then exhale for six through the lips. Only the hand on the stomach will rise or fall per time.

5. Taking the Calendar

"Patience is also necessary if you lose weight in a healthy and sustainable manner" does not need to get locked into a timeline if you work on meeting real goals, including taking 10,000 steps every day. New successes arrive every 24 hours; focus on them.

6. Identify your "Trouble Thinking"

Indicate the thinking that make you find yourself in trouble and work to stop and change them.' If you get nervous, or cravings. "Take them knowingly by saying' stop' clearly," it may seem dumb, but that simple action would break the chain of thought and give you the opportunity to bring you to a different, safer one.

7. Do not walk onto the scale

While the scale is not negative in nature, many of us have learned to equate it with self-destructive thoughts and actions. If you do this, don't even bother stepping down before you reach a place where the number on the scale doesn't determine. "The best way to do this is to count from one to 100 times you need until harmful feelings have gone away."

8. Forget the Whole "Foods Are Good or Bad" Mentality

Somewhere along the way, we tend to look or sound or proud of any choice we make. But it is just food, so you shoot. The expectations we set for ourselves are retribution, "and we would never bring our friends and loved ones to many of these standards.

9. Focus on the Attainable

"When you're not in the gym today, your target shouldn't be to go for 30 minutes on day one. A better goal could be to walk a 20-minute run," says researchers., "said researchers. "If you want to eat more, but you have no familiarity with healthy recipes, don't expect to make new healthy meals every night after work. Perhaps you should consider using a delivery service like HelloFresh, and Blue Stroke, where pre-portioned ingredients and recipes have been delivered at your door.

"THE MIND IS JUST LIKE A MUSCLE.

THE MORE YOU EXERCISE IT,

THE STRONGER IT GETS AND THE MORE IT CAN
EXPAND."

- Idowu Koyenikan -

Mindset Changes for Weight Loss

Pick every "diet" that you want. It will work in the short term, maybe. Yet make sure you have several coping approaches in your toolbox, which improve your chances of success. It will make a difference to tackle the physical, physiological, or behavioural dimensions of weight loss.

1. Know WHY you want to lose weight

What's the root of your inspiration, just how you want to lose weight? Want to lose weight before you date or get married? With the introduction of a time burden, short-term targets make weight loss even easier. This constant stress allows the stress hormone cortisol to rise, making it difficult to lose weight and may even increase the number on the scale. Shift your focus to you rather than lose weight for someone else. Want to lose weight in order to reduce the blood pressure? Perhaps it is painful for you to climb stairs and knee pain to bear the extra weight. Find out your WHAT. Find out the HOW.

2. Break up with your scale

Repeat. "I'm not a number." The existence of a category is both good and bad. It's useful as it gives you reviews. Only once a week (maximum) can you see if your weight has been lost and your weight loss stopped. More generally (even several times daily) weighting is problem-set, as weight fluctuations occur regularly because of such factors as water retention and glycogen storage levels.

The number of people becomes so injured that their everyday state determines. Sounds familiar? You know? A pound down? Yay! Yay! Yay! It'll be a wonderful day! A PUBLE? What even needs to be tried? I'll go eat a couple cookies then. Taking the scale and let the clothes show you exactly how you do. You will note that the taistband is a bit looser after about two weeks of healthy food. This is lead now!

3. Develop positive attitudes.

The diet and weight loss also correlate with negative feelings and fear of failure. When you are feeding, you tend to talk about everything you can't eat, and you have a feeling of hunger and lack too much mental energy. Switch this trend downside up and start to look at the glass as half-full, if it sounds familiar. Look at everything you can get nutritious and delicious food.

Rather than say, "I cannot eat that," say, "I plan to eat that. "How much better all becomes mood and touch. Start with simpler, easier-to-reach targets such as fruits instead of fried food and move to more aggressive priorities. Such smaller "winners" build your confidence and get you motivated to keep going. Encircle yourself also with those who inspire you, which is important in difficult times.

4. Have patience

It's impossible to lose 10 pounds overnight, as much as you would like. Shows such as The Biggest Loser and Extreme Makeover glorify large losses. Such tests don't sadly say you from which the weight was lost. When you lose weight, you lose a fat, water and muscle mix.

The goal is to preserve the structure of the muscles by maintaining strength and growing the dietary protein so that excess weight will mainly be caused by obesity. This can arise when gradual and steady weight loss happens. It's like the tortoise and the hare tale–the race wins steadily and endlessly. Therefore, the gradual loss of weight is more likely to remain a constant loss of weight.

5. Have a strategy

Researchers say, "If you don't prepare, you plan to fail! "Okay? The loss of weight is like a trip across the world. You need a roadmap on how to get from the beginning to the end. Take a couple of minutes each night to prepare your supper for the next day and workout. Once you prepare the meals and grab a refresher for the day ahead, you will not be able to take a treat, or visit the vendor, when the beast is horrific at 3 pm. And there are some road hazards and detours along the way, like every ride. Remember what you have experienced in the past (eating with friends, heat, sleepless nights) and finding alternatives for non-food. Journaling, listening to music, meditating, chatting to a stroll and a friend are some of the strategies that we recommend our clients try to deal with, rather than defaulting on chips or ice cream packets.

6. Write it down

A notebook that records your food, workout, attitude and appetite is one of the best tools to achieve success. A lot of tools are available to monitor your food and exercise, which is great because it will give you instant feedback on how you do it and on what you may need to do for tomorrow or the rest of the day. Will can find perspectives on your eating patterns, including some detail on your hunger level and your emotional health.

Should you feed only when you are hungry emotionally or if you feel sad, lonely, overwhelming or bored? Would you stop eating when you're half or max, no matter how much food sits on the plate? The citizens of Japan state that you only food up to 80 percent of them are full, namely Hara Hachi Bu. It takes between 15 to 20 minutes to get a message from your brain that you are filled and so avoids overfeeding and that awful sensation of being filled. This type of practice understands organically that it takes you Take every few bites to determine your hunger level at your next meal.

7. Don't equate yourself with other

Weight loses isn't a one-size-everything material. Perhaps what works for a person doesn't work. Meet with a certified nutritionist who specializes in weight loss to create a customized program. Every travel is special as each individual is built differently. And give it time. Give it time. Don't change your diet or exercise habits simply because someone else has been working well.

8. Do Yoga and Meditation

In your daily life, yoga and meditation stimulate the brain's consciousness and attention areas, which is good for keeping track of weight loss.

To order to cope with comfort eating or a binge, these behaviors often reduce the stress and improve gladness levels. It is easier to make the right choices when your mind is at ease.

"ONCE YOUR MINDSET CHANGES,

EVERYTHING ON THE OUTSIDE

WILL CHANGE ALONG WITH IT."

- Steve Maraboli -

Techniques That Work For Making A Sustainable Change In Your Diet

When they claim they want to lose 10 pounds or more, why can't a person succeed? The explanation for this is that they don't care about it ready to work for it. Your body won't respond if you're not prepared for your mind. It's so easy. You should get to the stage where your mind regulates your body and not the other way around to produce a real winning diet outcome. You must be strong mentally!

The week starts as you expect. You have adopted the diet by letter and started to see improvements. You know that this is the moment for you to actually achieve your goals.

Two weeks easily. It's a completely new story today. Rather than you would like to admit, you have lied on your diet plan and it's no longer totally on. You drown your sorrows in a Ben & Jerry pint, fed up and irritated. Maybe this culinary thing isn't just for you.

Hold it up. Hold it up. Your food isn't the issue here. It's your mindset–or habits, as is probably the case–about your food. You have a little chance of actually achieving results if you eat and try to change everything in your life at once. It's a change of mind that you really need here.

You need to stop looking for recipes and search for methods that you can use in your life. Think about it for a minute, it'll be betting if you go on a diet plan. You cook five rather than three times a day now and you sometimes eat that you have not been able to do before.

You're losing your two best friends on Friday night dinner because your diet won't allow you to dine at the restaurant. How do you ever expect to stay on the schedule with all this happening? This is clear. You're not going to.

If you want success, though, you have to stop focusing on this complete overhaul of all you learn and focus instead on building good habits, one by one. A tradition is something you do without thought immediately. Therefore, the more wise you make these choices, the better it will be to' stick' to them over time.

And you can dramatically increase the chances of success by choosing to focus on just one at a time (rather than a dozen). Studies in the field of social psychology has shown you to have a 85% chance of success if you add a new behavior change to your life and do so every day for 2-4 weeks? Or, if you make two changes in behavior to your life, the success rate declines to 35%. But now you can bank on less than 10% if you are super ambitionate and want to do three things at the same time.

Knowing the diet is all about shifting lifestyles and slowly developing habits. This is not a race (which will never come forward if you believe it's). Now, what can you do to make sure you look and see results? This is your strategy of five measures.

Phase 1: Choose a simple and straightforward to do.

First of all, choose a simple change that you can rely on. This move would include a piece of fruit for breakfast, for example, to help you fulfill your five to ten daily needs. Or, it could mean eating it a lot to figure out how much calories you have to consume every day. You can help to build your routines and achieve success by monitoring your intake.

Phase 2: Be alert for the difficult point of view.

Now, things will get complicated at some point during this process. Pretty rough. Be able to do so. Know that it will be better if you press on. You will probably experience some opposition, generally from 5-7 days, with every behavior change.

Phase 3: Take thought on or off.

The time has come to get rid of the misconception that this transition is temporary. When you change (or become used to it) this new lifestyle, start thinking about it to change the way you live your life forever. As you tend to consider it as something that lasts forever, the more quickly you erase from your mind the idea of potentially stopping.

Phase 4: Training, practicing and learning.

Practice as many times as possible this new habit. Repetition matters really and helps guarantee that you are effective in a healthy new habit. When you forget something once or twice, do not panic at the same time. You want to learn, not good.

Phase 5: Concentrate on your habits.

Would you like a trick to simplify things? Stop thinking about this transition and think about the things you're doing, instead. Concentrate on this and the others will collapse.

You eliminate the odds of getting overwhelmed if you see how high your long-term goal can be by doing it at once. Too many people feel like failing if they do not achieve the immediate gratification they want. But if you only work on day by day, you will know every day the feeling of success if you have completed what you have set out to do. So there are the five steps you can take on a regular basis to build some new habits and change your lifestyle.

...

YOUR HABITS BECOME YOUR VALUES,
YOUR VALUES BECOME YOUR DESTINY.

- Ghandi -

Ways to Ditch the Diet Mentality and Be Healthier

Forget your diet and the attitude of "mind what you eat." Choose a healthy way to eat and learn how to appreciate what your body can do.

Consider another solution that does not immediately assume that you need to limit your food choices and daily meals in order to become healthy.

Say you do not want to focus on a lot of dropping pounds, burning calories (or not consuming) or spending minutes every day. Rather, imagine eating your food, listening attentively and respecting your body's needs.

This year, make a decision to observe conscientious diet and exercise routine, without counting pounds or minutes to assess the success. You can just end up happier than you'd have been by beginning the same old culinary music and spinning again. You can only do that.

❖ Learn to Appreciate Fullness

Fullness is another emotion that can take some time to understand and respect. Diets advise you to eat a part or number of calories until you feel' good.' Nevertheless, the body has a normal way of regulating the intake of food and of meeting the needs for nutrients. When you're completed, the emotions and feelings of your body tell you; you just have to learn to listen.

Once you sleep enough and eat food you like, you begin to feel full and satisfied. Yet note the rule of reduction of returns: even the things you enjoy most will not be more tasty after some stage of intake, because you have gone past fulfillment and have started eating beyond your wants.

Be patient with food and snacks, with no distractions: no televisions, no computers, no books or ipads. Stay alone for some time if it works.

Take one bite and take a break and make sure you feel full. When you know you should encourage yourself to eat again early (when you feel hungry), you will easily end a snack, dinner or dessert.

❖ Eat and Feel Good

No "wrong," "good" or "evil" food is available in a cautious feeding. These are classifications and moral values that limit diets and decide how you behave about foods.

Instead, learn how to concentrate on food. You feel content as you start to eat your favorite foods, eat if you are thirsty, and stop eating if you are fully satisfied. If you eat a salad, a cookie, a fries ' sandwich, or a piece of fruit may be a matter of course.

If you eat attentively, it feels good to consider the needs of your body and your personal food habits. You did something to value yourself, not because you were playing by the rules.

❖ Move Mindfully, Too

Much Often you feel good working hard. It feels good to be outside or to have a stroll with a friend or partner. Sometimes. You might also skip some of your body's cues if you've put yourself limits on what "workout" is or what kind of "exercise" you do.

As you already are hungry and whole, start renouncing the rules of action. What rules determine what you do, how do you feel when you do it, what outcomes you get from it, whether you feel that a work-out applies only when it has a rough, sweating or one hour long time. This is also a diet, in other words.

Take care of what motivates you to work. Then step in the directions you like, which will give you a good feeling.

❖ **Pledge to Mindful Eating and Movement This Year**

Pledge to your mind this year to break the list of dietary rules, so change and respect your appetite and fullness. This year continues with the plan. Finally, experiment with different kinds of action you like.

It is a perfect year for you to reconsider' success' and whether you have succeeded in any diet or exercise routine you have attempted. Be more conscious of how diet and exercise make you feel, and love doing what you feel good, instead of limiting yourselves to rules and limits.

❖ Break Rules

Make a list of rules that you have to consider every day when, why, what and how much you eat. Pick one each week to break, or follow the list at a rate you feel at home. In this point, relying on an insightful and diligent food qualified registered dietitian is beneficial.

Start tuning into the signs of appetite and completeness of your body.

Be patient with this move if you have been on a diet for years (or decades) or have a history of trouble-like food. The body is used to hunger and fullness signs being overlooked, but all about beginning to feel, appreciate and enjoy them. It sounds easy, but it can be a challenge: when you start feeling hungry, honor that with a dinner or snack (depending on your daytime and hunger level).

In the beginning, the reaction to hunger may be to wonder, or to mistrust, "Why am I starving when I have lunch?" But just keep understanding it by encouraging yourself to feed before you become hungry.

When you become comfortable, it becomes harder to make conscientious food choices, such as irritability and difficulty concentrating. When you start eating when you feel hungry, you will enjoy your favorite food.

FOOD IS FUEL, NOT THERAPY!

- Life tracker -

Psychological Tips for Successful Weight Loss

Remember that you came back last week from a marriage that you wanted! Waiting eagerly for the pictures of your email, you get a set of people only for you to be even more frustrated! It looks like you must get into a weight loss program and finally push yourself! Then you think that for a very long time you were about to lose weight, but what stopped you?

We might like to shock you that even weight loss is correlated with a certain degree in psychology! No, this is certainly no disease, but there are certain rules, suggestions and strategies that dictate how much your weight loss plans can play out as soon as they arise.

1. Goal Settings

The first thing that comes to mind as we think about weight loss is to set a realistic goal. Before knowing where you want to go, you cannot begin a journey!

One of the key factors to lose weight is to realize how big a target is?

If your target is too far-reaching, it is going to fatigue you and you may want to leave before you get there. If your target is somewhat tame, your mind probably won't like to follow it, because the human mind has something to fight!

For eg, if 30 kg are overweight, according to your estimates, you will achieve an unsatisfactory result by setting a target of 45 kg, or a mere 5-8 kg.

It is best to choose a very daunting goal and send your unconscious mind a message of commitment, but not to the degree to which you lose interest and ultimately attempt to do so.

2. Patience

The hidden fact is that the effects of weight loss are not delivered in 30 minutes to you in comparison to your beloved fast food! It requires commitment, dedication, effort (both mental and physical), and nothing less perseverance (factor that motivates you to eat and to make unhealthy choices). It is still appropriate to slow down the weight loss cycle, but you're always effective. Results take time to prepare and the mind must not give up with a hat falling.

3. Liberty

The mind is a wonderful item–it's almost like a little boy! Regardless of your age, you'd like a break from the routine. So it may seem great that you have been able to get your readings down from time to time, but you will be encouraged by a little recompense. Of starters, if you want to lose 30 kgs, it is a little reward of your choosing that acts like a tension burst for your body and mind when you lose 5 kgs every day. However, it is your task to make sure you do not have the little kid (your brain) too much sugar to get your cavities! (Losses in results with weight loss)

4. Take Note

Remember that the most weight loss trainers neglect one of the tasks is that a daily journal or newspaper is important! Consider it the practice to reduce the exact amount of food and calories taken in each day, the quantity of water ingested (glass by glass or count tags) and the workout duration and intensity.

This helps your mind work in a tighter way when you record it, even though recording is for you. You are less likely to deviate from your approved program merely because you are afraid to "upload" them to your diary or journal.

5. Get that first step! Take that first step!

The launch of the weight loss plan is the most serious impediment of all the information given. One basic thing that actually helps you wake up and get ready is to continue with your weight loss regime. Ideally most people are afraid of getting dressed from the fitness center or a morning stroll, because of how it feels.

Nonetheless, you can change this by simply giving you a basic piece of advice–buy new track pants and shoes and make sure you enjoy color and style. Wear your trainers soon, sleep with your suit just as you get up out of bed. Then sit down and decide whether you want to go! The weight loss is hopefully very easy, unless you can decipher the mind's actions. (We can bet, you're sure will!) It is not really difficult when you try to internalize the improvements and strategies that may be required to modify the expectations of the brain.

Finally, note that your freedom is what you eat and it can either heal you or hurt you. It means you can make the right choice with your food, either with your medication or your poison.

Ways to Motivate Yourself to Lose Weight

It may sometimes seem difficult to continue and stick to a healthy weight loss program. Individuals also either lack the motivation to begin or lose their motivation to continue. Luckily, you can improve inspiration.

1. Determine why you want to lose weight

Clearly define and write down all the reasons for losing weight. It allows you to remain committed and motivated to achieve your weight loss goals. Try to read them every day to remind them of the weight loss plans you are trying to postpone.

Yours might be to avoid depression, stay up with grandchildren, search for a case, boost self-confidence or wear in a pair of jeans. Most people start to lose weight as a doctor has recommended it, but evidence shows that people are best off if their inspiration for weight loss comes from within.

2. Have Realistic Expectations

Most diets and food items say fast and easy weight loss. Have realistic expectations Many physicians prescribe that you lose just 1–2 pounds per week (0.5–1 kg).

Fixing unattainable targets will lead and cause you to give up feelings of frustration. Alternatively, it adds to a feeling of fulfilment to reach and accomplish achievable goals.

People who achieve their self-determined weight loss goals also have a higher chance of maintaining their weight loss in the long run. In a survey using details from several weight loss centers, the most likely out of the system is women who expected to lose the weight.

The good news is that only a slight loss of weight of 5–10% of your body weight will affect your health. When you're 82 kg (180 pounds), it's only just 4–8 kilograms. You're 250 kilograms, 13-25 kilograms (6-11 kilograms)

In addition, a loss of 5–10% of your body weight may:

- Increase blood suga control
- Lower cholesterol risk

- Decrease joint pain
- Reduce risk of certain cancers
- Reduce risk of cardiac disease

3. Focus on Process Goals

Most who try to lose weight and carry their targets or aims to reach at the end of the process. In fact, the final target weight will be an end objective.

Your drive can be undermined if you rely only on success expectations. Often you can feel too far away and feel exhausted.

You should instead describe project goals, or what steps you should take to achieve the desired results. Four days a week is an indication of a cycle target.

A study conducted by 126 overweight women in a weight loss program found that those who concentrate on the process are less likely than those who focuses on weight loss outcomes themselves to lose weight and are less likely to deviate from their diet.

Consider setting SMART targets in order to achieve clear objectives.

- SMART stands for:
- Specific
- Measurable
- Attainable
- Time-based

Some SMART targets include:

- I am going to walk quickly for 30 minutes five days next week. The same is the opposite.
- Every week I'm going to eat four portions of vegetables.
- This week, I'm just going to drink soda.

4. Pick a Plan That Fits Your Lifestyle

Choose a weight loss plan you can follow and keep away from plans that are virtually impossible to follow in the long term. Find a plan that fits your lifestyle. Although hundreds of diets are available, most are caloric-cutting.

Reducing your calorie intake can result in loss of weight, but diet, especially often Yo-yo, is a predictor of future weight gains.

Consequently, avoid strict diets that exclude certain foods entirely. Evidence also found that "all or nothing" people are less likely to lose weight.

Consider creating your own customized program instead:

- Reduced calorie consumption
- Reduced portion size
- Snack size cuts
- Reduced fried food and bowl
- Incl. fruit and vegetables

5. Keep a Weight Loss Journal

Self-monitoring is crucial to weight loss motivation and success. Research has found that people who track their food intake are more likely to lose weight and maintain their weight loss.

Nonetheless, you have to write down everything you eat to properly keep a food journal. It covers dinners, drinks and the sweets that you eat from the office of your boss. In your food journal you can also chart your emotions. This can help you identify certain foodstuff causes and help you find safe ways to manage them.

You may create food records or use a website or app on pen and paper.

All of them have proved successful.

6. Celebrate your victories

It is difficult to lose weight and celebrate all your milestones and be inspired. When you meet a goal, give yourself some credit. Social media or group blogs are great places to express and help your achievements. You will increase your drive if you feel pride in yourself.

In fact, try to label changes in behavior and not just a single amount on the graph. When you, for example, have achieved your target, take a bubble bath or schedule a fun evening with your friends for four days a week.

In fact, by praising yourself, you can further boost your motivation.

It is necessary, however, to choose suitable rewards. Stop enjoying food for yourself. Do stop benefits that are such costly that you're never going to buy it or so meaningless that you can have it regardless.

- Getting a manicure
- Going to a movie
- Buying a new running top
- Having a cooking class

7. Getting Social Aid

People must receive regular aid and positive feedback. Tell your friends and family your weight loss goals so they can help you fly.

A weight loss buddy is also helpful for many people. You should work together, take responsibility for each other and support each other throughout the process.

It may also be helpful to include your family, but make sure that other people, such as your parents, also support you. Consider joining a support group in turn. The support groups both in person and online have proved to be helpful.

8. Make a pledge

Research indicates that public engagement is more likely to achieve its targets. It will encourage you to be honest and inform others about the targets in weight loss. Tell your friends and family and even talk about social media posting them. The better your responsibility, the more individuals you share your goals.

9. Think and Talk Positively

Those who are positive and confident that they can achieve their goals tend to lose their weight. Optimistic think and talk. Think and talk Interestingly, it is more likely to be done by those who use "shift speak."

Shift talk makes comments about your contributions to behavioral changes, the reasons for them and the actions you take to reach your goals. And begin to discuss the loss of weight favorably. Sometimes, think about your actions and bring your thoughts clearly into practice.

Evidence on the other hand shows that people who spend a lot of time simply contemplating the weight of their goals are less likely to achieve their goal. This is regarded as a mental treatment.

You need instead to differentiate psychologically. In order to simulate your emotional state, take a few minutes to imagine hitting your goal and then waste some more minutes considering potential obstacles.

A 134 student research made them eat their nutritional targets emotionally or psychologically. Those who differ psychologically have a greater chance of behaving. We consumed less calories, did more exercise and ate less highly calorific food.

As you can see in this research, comparing minds is more inspiring, which contributes to more actions than intellectual relish, so that the brain is led to believe you have already achieved.

10. Plan for Challenges and Setbacks

Everyday stressors will always surface. Prepare for Problems and Breakdowns Finding ways to prepare and build proper coping skills will allow you to be inspired irrespective of life. Holidays, birthdays or celebrations will always be there. During work or with the children, there will always be stressors.

The solution and brainstorming of these future weight loss problems and failures is critical. You won't get off the bridge and lose motivation. For ease, many are turning to cooking. This can cause you to miss your weight loss targets quickly. It will not happen to you by developing proper coping skills.

However, studies have shown that people with a better way of coping with depression are losing more weight and holding it longer.

Consider using some of these methods to cope with stress:

- Exercise
- Practice square breathing
- Take a bath
- Go outside and get some fresh air
- Call a friend
- Ask for help

Remember to also plan for holidays, social events and eating out. You can research restaurant menus in advance and find a healthy option. At parties, you can bring a healthy dish or eat smaller portions.

11. Don't Aim for Perfection and Forgive Yourself

You do not have to be perfect for success and forgive yourself. You are less likely to achieve your targets if you have an "all or nothing" attitude. If you're too conservative, maybe you find that you've got to say, "I had a blackberry hamburger and fried beef for a snack, so I could have pizzas for dinner."

And you must not beat yourself if you make an error. Thoughts of self-defeat just inhibit your inspiration. Forgive yourself, too. Note that your success will not be spoiled by one mistake.

12. Learn to Love and Appreciate Your Body

We have consistently found that people who don't like their bodies are less likely to lose weight. Steps to change the perception of the body will help you lose weight and keep losing weight.

In fact, those with a better image of their body prefer to choose a diet that they can maintain and try out new behaviors that allow them to accomplish their goals.

- Exercises.
- Acknowledge what your body can do.
- Do something for yourself like acupuncture or manicure.
- Encircle you with positives.
- Stop comparing you with others, especially celebrities.
- Wear clothing you like and that suit you well.
- Check the mirror and say things that you like about yourself openly.

13. Find an Exercise You Enjoy

The following action will strengthen the body image. You're doing physical work is an important part of weight loss. It not only makes you burn calories but also increases your well-being. The best way to do this is to do exercise and to live. There are many different types of activities and it is important to explore various options to find one that you like. Take into account where you want to train. Would you rather be indoors or outdoors? Want to work out in a fitness center or in your own home?

Figure out also whether you want to work with a group or alone. Group classes are common and help motivate many people. But it's just as good to work out on your own if you don't like group classes.

Eventually, while you're busy, listen to music, and inspiration could be improved. People are also more likely to perform while listening to music.

14. Find a role model

You can be inspired to lose weight by getting a role model. You will, however, select the right form of role model to stay motivated. Holding your fridge on a picture of a supermodel won't inspire you across time. Alternatively, you can comfortably interact with a role model.

You will keep you inspired by having a nice and positive role model. Perhaps a friend who has lost a lot of weight and inspiration can be yours. They can also look for inspiring stories about people who have lost weight effectively.

15. Get a puppy dog

Puppy Dog can be the best following weight loss. In reality, studies show that a having a dog can help you to lose weight.

A Canadian survey of dog owners showed that dog owners walked over 300 minutes a week overall, while dog owners only exercised about 168 minutes a week on average.

Third, dogs are very helpful emotionally. Contrary to your buddy's job, dogs almost always look forward to physical activity.

The extra benefit has been shown to improve the overall health and well-being of animals. Higher cholesterol, decreased blood pressure and less symptoms of alienation and stress have been associated with it.

16. Seek professional help if needed

Don't feel reluctant to meet with a professional for help on how to lose your weight, if necessary. Those with more faith will lose more weight in their knowledge and abilities. This may involve finding a registered dietitian to show you how to exercise properly on certain foods or a physiologist for workouts.

Most would also like to be held accountable by a doctor.

If you still look for inspiration, consider finding a motivational coaching counselor or nutritionist who is trained to help people achieve their goals. Motivated to lose weight is important for the effectiveness of long-term loss of weight.

People find various motivating factors, so it is important to find out, in particular, what motivates you. Try to be versatile and to enjoy the small successes of your path to weight loss. And don't be afraid if necessary to ask for help. You will find and be inspired to reach the weight loss goals with the right tools and assistance.

THE HARDER YOU WORK FOR SOMETHING,

THE GREATER YOU'LL FEEL WHEN YOU ACHIEVE IT.

- Motti Vaion -

Tips for Developing a Winning Mindset on Your Diet

Look back to a time when you wanted something so bad you would have done something to do. You were ready to achieve the objective, and you were hindered by nothing.

Speak of your diet and training regimen now. Perhaps you bear any additional weight you know you cannot lose. In tandem with the world's best exercise program, you can have the best diet in the world, but unless You adhere to it, You will not see results. Your thought is one of the key factors in the effectiveness of a diet.

If you don't see the outcomes you wished for, ask yourself this critical question of thinking: am I applying my diet as I have done in the past to other challenges? Am I really all in the motions or just going through them?

You need to build the attitude that will offer you results to lose weight.

Here are the tips for a winning attitude to your diet.

1. Know why you're dieting: Write down the five main reasons you must get weight loss daily and become balanced before you hit your ideal weight. Understand why you're dieting. It will burn them and keep you on board. Why is it just as important for you to do this.

2. Expect to create the body of your dreams: standards are innate and can always be updated. Take the decision today to allow your dreams to grow. Search for the pictures you want on the poster board of newspapers and search every day for men with bodies. Create in your head this picture and predict it. It will get you to behave yourself in ways that contribute to your expected outcome.

3. Do have highest confidence: Do not feel bad because you are in the mainstream if you do not have self-confidence due to past mistakes. Decide today to grow up physically and get sick of it for 21-30 days. Your success will provide you with the courage to follow your next goal.

4. Make a commitment or die: test the degree of dedication to suit your last seven days actions. If you are not on the road to 100% conformity, forgive yourself and start today.

5. Use the determination power: define and write down five separate times in your life that you resisted before you succeeded. Read them for the next seven days every morning and immerse yourself in the consciousness that was required to persevere.

6. Build a team of supporters: no silence is required. Call three friends or family members nearest to you and invite them to be on your support team. It's easy to leave if you are alone, but it's a different story to let a team of people who matter about you down.

7. Return for implementation: For now, give yourself a small (non-food) treat when your diet and workout routine complies with 100 percent, and you know how it makes you feel. If it works, every day or at least once a week it will make new bonuses. You won't need incentives when the fight is over and the new habits are in place. Physically and mentally you'll feel so good that you'll wonder why you weren't ready before long.

8. Have a sense of urgency: make yourself ready now rather than later. Not next week. Not next week. Not after the heat. Not after your birthday. Do now, as long as time remains. Do it now, as long as you have a choice.

9. Get around people who support your goal: Make a decision to separate yourself from people who refuse to help you achieve your fitness goals. Your life is at stake, which needs drastic action. Just say no to spend time with people because they agree with your greatest goals and aspirations.

10. Never say die: agree you're going to do anything to match, and never say you're going to die. This is not a game. You're going to fight for weight and get sicker when you struggle. A rock solid determination is the only thing between you and the life of sickness and a future of plenty of health. Build your energy today and watch it soar.

Everything is possible if you have the mind, the will and the will to do so and to devote your time forward.

YOUR PROBLEM ISN'T THE PROBLEM,

IT'S YOUR ATTITUDE ABOUT THE PROBLEM.

- Ann Brashares -

Common Mistakes to Avoid When Choosing Weight Loss Diets

Every year, weight loss diets are decided by people. It's usually part of a plan for the New Year. Though, most people make the mistake of choosing the wrong diet and end up losing weight all year round. That is why it is so important to choose the best weight loss diet.

You want to make sure you choose the right diet this time. Nonetheless, you may not be exactly how to choose with all the weight loss diets available. Okay, when people select diets, a number of common errors occur. Let's see and how you can stop these errors. You are more likely to choose the right diet if you prevent these common mistakes.

Mistake 1: A diet with <u>False promises</u>: One major error that people make when selecting from all the possible diets to reduce weight is a diet that makes false statements. Within one month, some diets claim to help you lose 40 pounds. This is crazy, and even if it sounds great for you, it's not a diet for which you should be using it.

Another false argument that weight loss diets make is that without doing anything you can lose a lot of weight. Without certain causes, overweight does not exist. By making changes, you will be unable to lose weight. Don't make this common error if you want to choose a plan for weight loss.

Mistake 2: <u>Absolutely leaving out a diet</u>: An other common error is selecting a diet that completely cut out a food group when considering a diet for weight loss.

The equilibrium is important for your body. You should not strip out a full category of foodstuffs. Naturally, you should minimize any calories to help you lose weight.

Most plans for weight loss depend on completely cutting out carbs or you don't want to consume any fats. This might not be the healthiest solution. Your body needs a healthy dietary intake. It is a challenge to cut back, but it is probably a bad decision to completely eliminate one product or another. You're probably not going to adhere anyway to this kind of diet.

Mistake 3: <u>No Exercise Diet</u>: Choosing weight loss diets without a schedule for exercise is also a big error. To lose weight, you will burn off calories. You're not going to lose if you don't burn off calories. It's not necessary to minimize what you consume. Exercise is important in order to lose weight in a healthy way, so do not make a mistake and go for an diet with no exercise.

Mistake 4: <u>Paying Hugely Huge money for a diet plan</u>: The common fault when selecting weight loss diets is that you pay huge money for a diet plan. The budget should not be violated by a good diet schedule. Many diets only want people who desperately lose weight to gain money. Do not let people exploit you in this way. By spending a huge sum of money, you will lose weight.

It is important to avoid these mistakes when choosing diets for weight loss. You will make a good choice as long as you avoid them. Hold these mistakes in mind when looking at the diets for weight loss to help make you lose fat from the body. You should make a good choice to remove the extra pounds.

Best Ways to Maintain Weight Loss

Unfortunately, even people losing weight ultimately recover it. In fact, only about 20 percent of dietitians who start with weight lose weight and keep it off on a long-term basis. But don't let you dissuade this. There are a few ways you can keep weight off, from stress management to stress control. You are scientifically proven.

Such techniques can be just what you need to provide numbers for you and keep your weight loss hard-won.

❖ **Note exercise**

Regular exercise also plays a major role in the management of weight. It can help you consume some additional calories and improve your metabolism, two things necessary to achieve an energy balance. If you're in the center of your nutrition, you're using the same amount of calories. This is more likely to keep the weight even.

Several studies have demonstrated that those with mild physical activities at least 200 minutes a week (30 minutes a day) following weight loss are more likely to remain weighty. In some cases much higher levels of physical activity may be required to maintain weight effectively. One study found that one hour per day of exercise is best suited for those who try to keep weight loss.

It should be remembered that walking in tandem with other lifestyle changes, including commitment to a healthy diet is most conducive to maintaining weight.

❖ **Eat breakfast Everyday**

Eating breakfast will help you achieve your weight maintenance goals. Breakfast eaters tend to have overall healthier habits, such as the use of more fruit and micronutrients and drinking more. In fact, breakfast eating is one of the better habits reported by people who handle weight loss effectively.

A study found that 78% of 2 959 persons who sustained a weight loss of 30 pounds (14 kg) for at least one year reported eating breakfast every day.

However, although people eating breakfast seem very good at sustaining weight loss, there are conflicting facts. Reports don't explain the inevitable weight gain or worse eating habits by missing the meal. Skip breakfast can potentially help some people meet their weight loss and maintenance aims.

This could be one of the things the individual does.

You will certainly have to do it if you believe like eating breakfast is important to your objectives. Nevertheless, if you're not happy to eat breakfast or if you don't hunger in the morning, skipping is free.

❖ **Eat Protein**

A lot of protein eat can help maintain the weight as protein can help lower hunger and encourage completeness. Protein raises levels of certain body hormones which are essential for weight control and cause satiety. A protein reduction in hormone levels which increase hunger has also been shown.

The effect of protein on your hormones and fullness will automatically reduce your daily calories, a major factor in weight maintenance. Protein also requires considerable energy to decompose the body. So it can increase the number of calories you burn during the day by consuming it daily.

On the basis of several studies, the impact of protein on metabolism and appetite tend to be most pronounced when about 30% of protein calories are used. In a calorie-diet it is 150 grams of protein.

❖ Weigh Yourself Regularly

Controlling the weight periodically by standing on the scale may be a helpful tool in weight maintenance. This ensures that it can warn you about your success and foster action in weight control.

When you weigh yourself, your mind say you to eat less calories all day, which is good for weight loss. For one study the weight of the individuals six days a week was, on average, 300 fewer calories a day than the weight of those who tracked less often. How many times is a personal choice to measure yourself. Many people find it helpful to test their weight once or twice a week, while others do so more effectively.

❖ Be Mindful of Your Carb Intake

When you pay attention to the forms and volume of carb you ingest, it may be easier to maintain the Carb intake. It can be detrimental to your weight maintenance targets to eat too many refined carbs, including white soup, white pastes and fruit juices.

Such foods have been separated from the natural fiber needed to promote completeness. Fiber-low diets are associated with hypertension and weight gain. You may also help maintain your weight loss by reducing your carb intake total. Some studies found that in some circumstances, weight is more likely to be kept away in the long term by those who adopt low-carb diets following weight loss.

Furthermore, the risk of people eating more calories than they expend is greater for the weight maintenance with the low-carb diet.

❖ Lift Weights

A common adverse effect of loss of weight is a decreased muscle mass. It can decrease the weight, because muscle loss reduces the appetite, and you eat less calories all day long.

If you do some form of resistance training like weight lifting, your muscle will be stopped and your metabolism will be maintained or even increased. Studies show that weights are more likely to be raised following weight loss while maintaining muscle mass.

It is recommended that you take physical training at least twice a week to obtain these advantages. Both muscle groups should work toward optimal results in your training system.

❖ Be Prepared for Setbacks

At least, on your weight maintenance path Setbacks are possible. Occasionally you give in or skip a workout. There may be days when you do. Nonetheless, a slip up sometimes doesn't mean that you should chuck your goals away. Just go ahead and make better choices.

It can also help plan situations in the future that will make eating healthy, such as a birthday or a wedding, challenging for you.

❖ Keep to Your Diet All Week Long (Even on the week-ends)

The habit of eating healthfully on weekdays and "cheating" on the weekends is one that also leads to weight loss. Many people are driven to junk food, which can substitute for efforts to maintain weight. this mentality. You will gain more weight than in the first place, if it becomes a regular habit. Conversely, evidence has shown that weight loss is more common for those who observe a healthy diet schedule all week long.

One study found that, relative to those that allowed more autonomy on weekends, individuals were almost twice as likely as those who retained their weight in less than a year (2,2 kg) in a weekly coherence.

❖ Stay Hydrated

For some reasons, drinking water is beneficial to maintain weight. This encourages completeness first and can help you regulate your calories whether you consume one or two glasses before meals.

For one study, people who have drank water before eating a meal have 13% less calory consumption than people who have not taken water. In fact, the number of calories you eat during the day was shown to increase slightly.

❖ Get enough Sleep

Getting enough sleep has a significant impact on weight control. Getting sufficient sleep. In fact, sleep deprivation seems to be a significant risk factor for gaining weight in adult people and can interfere with maintaining weight.

This is partially because poor sleep leads to higher levels of ghrelin, dubbed the' starving hormone,' since it makes people feel more attractive.

However, weak sleepers tend to have lower leptin levels, a hormone that is needed to control their appetite.

In fact, sleepers are simply tired and less driven to train and make good food choices, for short periods of time.

Find a way to change your sleep habits if you don't get enough. It is good for weight control and overall health to cycle for at least seven hours a night.

❖ Managing stress levels

Stress management is an important part of weight control. In addition, the increased amount of cortisol which is an hormone released to respond to the stress will lead to weight recovery.

Higher amounts of belly fat, large appetite and food consumption are related to consistently higher cortisol. Stress is also a common source of impulsive eating, even if you are not hungry while you eat.

Luckily, you can do many exercises to combat tension, such as diet, yoga and meditation.

❖ Look for a support system

Achieving your weight goals alone can be challenging. One way to overcome that is to consider a support system to keep you accountable in your healthy lifestyle and likely to work with you.

A series of studies have shown that it can be helpful if a friend has a similar healthy habits as a partner or wife to achieve your goals. Another study analyzed the health habits of more than 3000 people and found the other more likely to follow their example while another person is living a healthy habit, including exercise.

❖ Track Your Food Intake

A Monitor Your Food intake is a more effective way to maintain weight loss for those who monitor their intake of food in a diary, an online food log or an app. Food trackers are useful as they raise awareness about how much you consume, as they often offer specific information about the number of calories and nutrients that you use.

Some food monitoring apps allow you to monitor your workout so that you can guarantee that your weight is preserved.

❖ **Eat plenty of plants**

Multiple studies relate high intake of vegetables to better control of weight. Vegetables are low in calories in the beginning.   You should eat large portions without weight loss while still eating a lot of nutrients.

In fact, vegetables are high in fiber and can potentially reduce the number of calories you eat during the day, thereby increasing the sense of fullness. Try to eat one to two servings of vegetables for each meal for these weight control effects.

❖ **You have to be Consistent**

Coherence is essential to weight control. It's better to stick to your new healthy diet and lifestyle instead of on - and-off eating finishing in switching to older habits. When you first adopt a new "way of life," making healthy decisions is second nature if you are comfortable with them. It can be daunting.

You will be effortless in your healthy lifestyle, so that you can keep your weight even better.

❖ **Practice Mindful Eating**

Mindful cooking is the practice of listening to internal hunger signals and paying full attention during the meal cycle. This means slowly feeding without distractions, and carefully chewing food, so that you can feel the scent and flavor of your meal.

You will most likely stop feeding when you're really finished when you eat this way. It may be difficult to recognize fullness if you consume while you are overwhelmed, and you may end up eating more. Careful diet studies show that weight maintenance is beneficial when reducing habits commonly linked to weight gain, such as emotional eating.

Therefore, those who eat attentively can retain their weight without calories counting.

❖ **Make Healthy Changes to Your Lifestyle**

The reason why a great many people fail to maintain their weight is that they follow unhealthy, long-term diets. We end up feeling depressed, which often leads to more weight loss than we lose as they return to normal.

Holding weight loss will change your lifestyle sustainably.

This is different for everyone, but it basically means that it is not too rigid, clear and safe decisions as often as possible. Diets can be restrictive and impractical, frequently contributing to weight loss.

Nonetheless, you can adjust your pattern quickly to retain your weight loss in the long term. There are a lot of simple adjustments. You should know that your weight control requires much more than what you eat during your ride. Fitness, sleep and mental health also have a role to play.

Maintenance of weight can be easier if you just take a new way of living instead of trying and avoiding weight loss.

WHEN YOU GIVE THE SUPPLY OF DISCIPLINE,

LIFE BECOMES EASY FOR YOU.

- Sunday Adelaja -

The Best Diet Plans: Sustainability, Weight Loss and More

Nearly half of adults are expected to try and lose weight every year. Changing your diet is one of the easiest ways to lose weight. But, because you are not sure which diet is most appropriate, safe and efficient, the strictly available food plans make it difficult to get going. Many diets are designed to reduce your hunger for food, while others recommend reducing your use of calories and carbohydrates or fat.

Furthermore, others deliver safety benefits that go beyond weight loss. These are the best diet strategies for weight loss and overall health changes.

1. Intermittent fasting

Intermittent fasting is a food technique that works from time to time. There are various forms, including a 16/8 approach that decreases calorie consumption to 8 hours per day, and a 5:2 system that reduces calorie consumption to 500–600 calories twice per week every day.

How it works: Intermittent fasting reduces the time to eat. This is a simple way to reduce your calorie consumption. This can lead to a loss of weight, except for the moment you are supposed to consume too much sugar.

Weight loss: Intermittent rapidity has been shown to cause a weight loss of 3–8 percent over a 3-24 week period in a research analysis. The same study found that this form of ingestion would decrease the diameter of the tail by 4–7%, a proxy for unhealthy bowel fat.

Many studies have found that intermittent fasting can maximize fat consumption while preserving muscle mass that can increase metabolism.

Other advantages: transient rapidity has been correlated with anti-aging effects, increased sensitivity to insulin, enhanced brain health, reduced inflammations and many more.

Downsides: For most healthy adults, intermittent fasting is usually safe. Sensitive individuals to decreases in blood sugar levels, like some people with diabetes, low weight, or an eating disorder, should speak to a healthcare professional prior to beginning intermittent fasting, as well as women pregnant or breastfeeding.

2. Plant based diets

Plant based diets can help you lose weight. Plant based diets The most common forms are vegetarianism and veganism that constrain animal products for reasons of health, ethics, and the environment. There are, however, also more versatile herbal diets such as a flexitarian diet, which is a herbal diet that gradually requires animal products to be consumed.

How it works: There are many forms of vegetarianism, but they are mostly beef, poultry and fish excluded. Eggs and milk can also be avoided by some vegetarians.

The vegan diet takes it a step further by reducing the number of animal products and items of animal origin such as butter, gelatin, honey, whey, casein and albumin.

The flexitarian diet does not fall under clear rules, as this is not a diet, but a lifestyle change. This allows most people to eat bananas, vegetables, legumes and whole grains, but it offers a mild complement to proteins and animal products. Many of the limited food classes contain high calories, which can help to reduce the loss of weight.

Weight loss: Evidence has shown that weight loss in herbal diets is successful. A survey of 12 studies involving 1,151 students revealed that total plant diet losses in animal products were 4.4 pounds (2 kg).

However, after a vegan diet, people who did not eat a diet on vegetables lost an Average of 5.5 pounds (2.5 kg). Plant-based diets can also help you lose weight, as they appear to be high in nutrients, which can help you stay healthy and have low calorie content.

Additional benefits: Plant-based diets have been related to several other advantages, such as a low risk of chronic conditions such as heart disease, tumors and diabetes. These can also be safe more economically than meat-based diets.

Downsides: While herbal diets are safe, essential nutrients usually found in animal products such as magnesium, vitamin B12, vitamin D, calcium, zinc and omega-3 fatty acids can also be decreased.

3. Low-carb diets

One of the most common diets for weight loss is low-carb diets. The atkins diet, ketogenic diet (keto) and low carbide, high fat diet (LCHF) are some examples. Many animals drastically decrease their carbon dioxide. Of example, diets with very low carbs like keto are less than 10 percent of the total calories for this macronutrient, compared with less than 30 percent for other types.

How it works: Low-carb diets minimize the intake of protein and fat in your carb. These are typically more protein-intensive than fat diets which are important, because protein can lead to appetite reduction, metabolism increasing and muscle mass retention. The body begins to use fatty acids instead of energy sources in very low-carb diets such as keto by storing it in ketones. The ketosis is known as this operation.

Low-carb diets can support weight loss and can be more effective than traditional low-fat diets. A survey of 53 experiments with 68,128 participants, for example, found that low-carb diets lead to significantly increased weight loss compared with low-fat diets.

However, low-carb diets seem quite successful when unhealthy bowel fat is combusted.

Certain advantages: Evidence shows that low carbon diets can reduce heart disease risk factors, including elevated cholesterol and blood pressure. For people with type 2 diabetes, it can also raise blood sugar and insulin levels.

Downsides: LDL (bad) cholesterol may be elevated by a low carb diet in some cases. Really low-carb diets can also be hard to follow and can cause some people stomach problems.

In rare cases, ketoacidosis can cause a dangerous metabolic syndrome that is fatal if left untreated with a very low-carb diet.

4. The paleo diet

The paleo diet is the same foods the parents are thought to have consumed. It is based on the theory that contemporary ailments are related to the west diet, although supporters claim that the human body has not transformed into legumes, grains and milk.

How it works: The Paleo Diet encourages the intake of whole meals, berries, plants, maggot foods, nuts and seeds. This bans food consumption, fruit, sugar and milk, while a few less stringent forms require other milk products, such as cheese.

Weight loss: Several studies show that the paleo diet can help lose weight and reduce the amount of unhealthy fat in the body. For instance 14 healthy adults lost average of 5.1 pounds (2.3 kg) during their palaeo diets in the 3-week test, and decreased by a total of 0.6 inches (1.5 cm) the circumference of their waist— proxy for belly fat. Research suggests, more than common diets like a Mediterranean diet and a low-fat diet, that paleo diets are more compressive. This can be because of its high content of protein.

Some benefits: After the paleo diet, risk factors such as high blood pressure, cholesterol and triglyceride may be decreased by several heart disease causes.

The paleo diet does, however, eliminate various food classes, including legumes, whole grains and cheese, while it is balanced.

5. Low-fat diets

Fatty, low-carb diets have been popular for decades, as are low-carb diets. A low-fat diet typically limits the intake of fat to 30 percent of your daily calories. Many high-and moderate-fat diets aim at reducing carb use to below 10% of calories.

How it works: Fat-free diets limit fat intaking, as fat contains approximately twice as many calories as the other two-protein and carbicians-macronutrients. Ultra-low-fat diets contain less than 10% fatty calories, with some 80% carbohydrate calories, and 10% protein calories. Ultra-low-fat diets mainly consist of meat and animal products based on plants and limitations.

Low-fat diets can aid with the loss of weight by reducing calorie intake.

An study of 33 trials of over 73,500 participants showed that small but significant improvements in weight and waist circumference have been observed with a low fat diet. While low-fat diets tend to be as effective as low-carb diets in controlled situations for weight loss, low-carb diets seem more effective everyday.

Ultra-low-fat diets, especially among people with obesity, have proven successful. An 8-week analysis of 56 people show, for example, that eating a 7-14% fat diet resulted in an average weight loss of 14.8 pounds (6.7 kg).

Some advantages: low fat diets have been associated with a decreased risk of heart disease stroke. It can also reduce inflammation and improve diabetes markers.

Downsides: Too much fat deficiency will lead to long-term health issues as fat plays an essential role in hormone production, absorption of nutrients and cell health. In comparison, very low fat diets were associated with an increased risk of metabolic syndrome.

6. The Mediterranean diet

The Mediterranean diet is based on foods consumed by persons in countries such as Italy and Greece. While designed to reduce the risk of heart disease, numerous studies suggest that weight loss can also be beneficial.

(I think I will soon make a book about one of the longest-running places in Italy and their typical foods, stay tuned!)

How it works: The Mediterranean diet is in favour of consuming lots of fruits, vegetables, nuts, seeds and legumes as well as tubers. Meat, eggs and milk products, such as chickens, must be consumed in moderation. Red meat is reduced in the meantime. Moreover, refined grains, Trans fats, fried oils, processed meats, added sugar and other high-processed foods are limited to the Mediterranean diet.

Weight loss: Although this is not necessarily the diet of weight loss, several studies have shown that a Mediterranean diet can help weight loss. An review of 19 trials, for example, found that people with a variation of the Mediterranean diet with a decrease in exercise or calories expended on mean 8.8 pounds (4 kg) more than the control diet.

Additional benefit: The Mediterranean diet contains a lot of rich foods with antioxidants that can help fight inflammation and oxidative stress by free radicals neutralization. The risk of heart disease and premature death was reduced.

Downsides: Since the Mediterranean diet is not a diet for loss of weight, people may not lose weight because they eat fewer calories.

7. WW (Weight Watchers)

WW is one of the world's most popular services for weight loss.

Although no food group is excluded, WW participants have to eat regularly to achieve their ideal weight within their specified areas.

How it works: WW is an ingredient-based system with a calorie, fat and fibre-dependent meaning on different foods and drinks. You must stay under your daily allowance to achieve the desired weight.

Weight loss: There are several studies that show that WW makes you lose weight. Across 45 trials, for example, participants on WW diets shed 2,6% of weight compared to those who sought regular therapy. In comparison, people who follow WW plans, compared to people who follow another programs, have been more effective in sustaining weight loss in several years.

Certain advantages: WW requires versatility to be implemented quickly. It allows people with food conditions and allergies to stick with the schedule.

Downsides: WW can be pricey based on the subscription plan, thus providing versatility. Often, if dietary staff prefer unhealthy foods, versatility can be downfall.

8. The DASH diet

The DASH lifestyle approach to preventing hypertension or DASH diet is a regimen that helps treat or avoid the clinically-known high blood pressure. This stresses the consumption of a great many fruits, vegetables as well as whole grains and lean meats.

Although the DASH diet does not represent a diet of weight loss, many people report weight loss.

The DASH diet advises certain portions of different food classes.

How it works: The amount of portions to consume is dependent on your daily consumption of calories. A DASH diabetic will eat about 5 portions of fruits, 5 portions of fruit, 7 portions of healthy carbs like whole grains, 2 portions of low-fat dairy products and 2 portions or less of lean meats per day, for example. Therefore, you should eat 2-3 days a week of nuts and seeds.

Loss of weight: The DASH diet can help lose weight. Reports have shown A survey of 13 research results, for example, found that the DASH diet was significantly lower than those on a placebo diet in 8-24 weeks.

Specific advantages: The DASH diet has shown a decrease in blood pressure and multiple risk factors for heart disease. It can also reduce your risk of breast and colorectal cancer and help fight recurrent depressive symptoms.

Downsides: While DASH can help with the loss of weight, the consumption of salt and blood pressure are mixed. Furthermore, consuming too little salt is linked to increased resistance to insulin and an elevated risk of mortality in people with heart disease.

You can lose weight with many diets. Some of the most common diets and meal programs include intermittent fasting, vegetative diets, diets that are low in carbs, low-fat diets, paleo dipping, the Mediterranean divertisement, WW and the DASH diet. While all of the above diets are proven effective in weight loss, it must be your lifestyle and dietary preferences that depend on your decision. It makes sure you stick to it more effectively on a longer term basis.

Weight Loss Through The Power Of Positive Thinking

Many want to lose weight and try the effects constantly, because they feel like they're on a roller coaster. In light of the myriad diets, it seems like the weight has been decreased or the findings have been misleading.

One of the key reasons why so many people try to lose weight is that they start the process with an expectation of disappointment rather than achievement. Even when the thought isn't necessarily negative, both preparation and the setting of targets, which is necessary for reaching every achievement in life, are still lacking confidence.

I once heard a gentlemen say something very profound, I remember. He did not quote him and simply said that everyone could do anything while they were ready to step outside their comfort zone slightly. Many people can learn to play guitar, for example, but many don't because they don't leave the comfort zone.

In reality, it takes one hour or even half an hour a day in this situation to go beyond the comfort zone, in this case work. This needs to be done. Just constant, not much.

Just as learning a new instrument or technique, it will take a step outside the comfort zone to lose weight. Unfortunately, the fight is lost before it begins as it was buried in misery in the mind. A idea creeps in the same way that the death klasse of a meal is ringing: "I've tried several diets and nothing works for me." The mind will work for us or against us. The mind is a powerful instrument. Have you ever met someone to warn everyone with complete confidence that they're going to get sick when cold and flu season arrive? And, in short, really, they get sick of cold or grippe?

Thinking like this is not only counter-productive to make progress in every effort; it is also harmful in its consequences for interpersonal relationships, coping capacity and self-image. Such forms of thoughts are diet killers and weight gain fillers for the person trying to lose weight.

How are we going to think then? This is by far the biggest challenge and still the most strong weapon in the battle of the bulge, which so many want to conquer. Shift your mind. Change your thinking. Concentrated and concentrated actions will be expected. This takes just as much preparation as playing guitar or becoming a professional artisan.

If the negative thoughts come into your head, replace them with positive thoughts that encourage and support them immediately. Don't think about the number of diets you have tried and failed, but about your success. Together with audibly positive statements, indulge in positive self-speak. Speak for yourself, in other words, confidently, and speak out clearly about yourself, saying what you are trying to achieve and motivating yourself. You and your condition must be special to them, which you can only think about. But, to provide an idea like "I'm happy I'll lose the weight" or "I'm strong and confident and I'll achieve my target." They're generic so they provide the kind of thought to execute.

In the skill you are able to conquer and rise high, there will be mental stress, physical effort, and emotional battles; particularly as you repeat these every day, out for several minutes and take part with everyday tasks.

When a human repeats an action for 30 days every day, he's gotten a habit. You'll have changed your perspective if you stick with your visible statements for ninety days.

Keep in mind that this optimistic, balanced and upward shift of mindset won't lose weight until sedentary patterns and diets are modified. Clearly, it is necessary to get up and move, from cycling to a rigorous physical fitness programme. The key point here is to train the mind for body control. Take the flesh to the moment.

When you understand your diet, you should not focus on food that causes negative effects, talk about what, when and the way you consume instead of the fun improvements. It promotes a more constructive way of thought. It is inspiring and optimistic to take on the challenge of weight loss and to adopt a new diet and exercise lifestyle. The search is filled with various recipes and methods of cooking, including new things and even tastes.

It is most rewarding to be more confident and self-confident in this entire process. Why does this happen? Depending on these positive attributes, you're changing how you think. In fact, shifting the diet to healthy foods full of nutrients and vitamins such as fresh fruits, raw vegetables and somewhat steamed vegetables, will improve overall health and wellness.

Clearly there are many other considerations that must also be taken into account before undertaking some type of exercise and diet. Every person is different and has a number of unique circumstances. Taking on the optimistic challenge, but do it with good research and training and ask your doctor or nutritionist questions in order to make sure you do the best for yourself. Hold something very critical in mind in relation to other people; for all that you do in life is good, my beloved sister used to call "power vampires." "Negative Nillies" I have always called them. Remember that you don't let them take the thunder; stay on track, stay positive and remain outside the comfort zone; that's the point. Live happily, sleep and be really well.

ALWAYS TURN A NEGATIVE SITUATION

INTO A POSITIVE SITUATION.

- Michael Jordan -

Enlisting Your Mind in the Battle of Weight Loss

You will not be one of those people who fail in thinking that weight loss is all physical before beginning the weight loss regimen. In reality, it is as much a physical mental battle as it is. And believe it or not, whether you win or lose the battle against unnecessary pounds, can your mind say. Here are some tips on how to change your attitude and lose the weight you want.

Take your time and relax and see what's the best way to lose weight for you. After your weight loss goals have been met, you can use the right motivation to keep focused. Motivation can mean various things, so it will be highly individual to different people. Mostly, though, it is your incentive to want to lose weight and begin with ONE THING.

Were you aware of a specific weight loss goal? The goal can be to attain a certain amount of pounds, to meet a dress size or just a general understanding of the ideal weight for which you shoot. You will judge if they are practical until you know just what your goals are. If you have set ambitious targets, you would probably make some unhealthy choices in trying to achieve them. You want to stay healthy while you are losing weight.

You will be frustrated when the time comes to achieve that goal if the goals you have set are impractical. For your thought, it can be catastrophic. Consider carefully before setting the goals. On the other side, if you set realistic targets, you will be able to succeed.

Find friends and families who support and encourage you in your attempts to lose weight as you focus on your emotional weight loss game. You need a reliable person that you can expect to be there if you are tempted or just need to speak to someone when you have a food or health problem.

It is highly likely that you will have a schedule as part of your weight loss journey. When you execute your schedule every day, create a system of rewards that will enable you to proceed. A low-fat smoothie with your choice fruit in it is one concept of a treat. It is critical that you choose something for which you are willing to work, but that the intent of the practice plan is not split and removed.

It is vital that you imagine yourself in your lower weight while you're starting your weight loss game. The explanation is that you are inspired to remain engaged in the system. If appropriate, find your dress to suit in the style you like and hang your dress in your bathroom or kitchen to assist you in visualizing this aim. You might also want to take pictures or even use a lower-weight version of yourself. Be sure to put your mental inspiration into the position you can see every day, whatever it takes.

When your attitude is right, it will be much easier for you to lose weight. Use these to get your program started now!

The Mind Also Matters in Healthy Living

Healthy living isn't just canned fruit and vegetables, fried and processed food is left untouched and every other day is reached by the gym. It's about developing a healthy mind too. Healthy life actually begins with a healthy mind.

❖ **Get your mentality right**

Anyone who ever tries to commit to a diet or an exercise regime would believe that the mind actually rules over the body is true to the old saying. There are no many who do not learn about vices such as smoking and drinking and healthy living values are good, healthy eating and exercising regularly. Nonetheless, there are numerous people who don't have the spirit to comply with these laws.

Here are some rules to help you win the game of your mind:

❖ **Do not be allowed to rule the weighing scale**:

Losing weight and maintaining the ideal body weight are usually two of your key healthy living targets. Nonetheless, this does not mean you can let out the burden on the weighing scale. Alternatively, you should send out messages that you feel better when you get up in the morning, raise your energy levels when changing to a new routine, and do less when embarking on a new diet program, or calculate your health and fitness levels for you.

❖ **Find a way to deal with stress other than by eating:**

Stress is an inherent part of our daily lives, so it doesn't really support your healthy living efforts to get through it. In the clouds, count blessings when you're feeled lousy, or take good readings, put some music you enjoy, or stroll around in the park when you're concerned about, there are countless different ways to cope with pain. These are ways to educate the mind in something else than rice.

❖ **Egg yourself.**

To avoid losing that level of motivation, make sure you're looking with realistic goals-I'll put in my old jeans by the end of two months and NOT "I'll lose 10 pounds for the next 4 days." For starters, if you've just got to cram in the pair of jeans at the end of the two months, don't mop it, but instead persuade yourself you are on the right path and you'll hit your target in no time.

❖ **Mental and rational**

Healthy living means creating an ambitious positive attitude when the odds are small and confident enough to listen and direct the body towards healthy living targets that suit you rather than what the book says.

Can You Open Your Mind Enough To Find True Weight Loss Success

It's often the issues that we have to contend with the most-if you are fighting against it, take note of it and make a conscious decision to investigate it more specifically. What we are fighting, too, persists. Therefore, to learn how to let things go is one of the best ways of overcoming internal opposition.

Most of us assume we know what is the problem (Too much fat? Not enough exercise?), and believe that we know what to do. But sometimes, assuming that we know the answers, we lose sight of the real problem or skip the multi-faceted problem.

Another explanation is that it so often does not work for approaches that' worked in the past. If we make several improvements together, we get benefits for several reasons. In addition we can see what we feel is the most significant positive factor, and relate it to all the tests. We conclude that we have' confirmation bias.

We think we are now mindful of the reaction, and we need to do it again to achieve results. But it is highly likely that something else, something darker, is the true issue, if you can not execute or if you are constantly' trying' and' failing. Even if it was not the first time that life progresses and it may not act in the future, what worked in the past.

Rarely is there a single cause, so there is seldom a single "solution." It is therefore important for us to open our minds to things we consider to be trivial. Often the "magic" lies in the small things!

The real aim of holistic health is to have a balanced approach and to incorporate all aspects of our lives. If any area is out of control, it's going to affect the others. We might focus on one or two aspects, but we are not even mindful of the limiting element. We need food, diet, health, emotional well-being, mental well-being, satisfaction, connections between people and stress management-but all these issues are too often overlooked or, worse, made harder when we want to make these physical changes!

So if we get stressed, we can get this on the nearest and dearest-so we hide from our marriages-because we eat too little and exercise too much. That cycle would make it harder only to lose the weight, as our hormonal system gets interrupted, and also when we feel stressed and feel emotionally under-par, we will have to exercise or diet well or prepate our food more. This often happens in binge diets or yo-yo diet, and we certainly don't make good, happy people!

Many of us believe like we excel because we shed body fat at fast speeds or run into the dirt and practice super-strict eating habits and obedience to our bodies. But in most situations, once we analyze the' real' progress it produces outcomes and actually keeps them. This develops new life habits and attitudes that make us content in our own skin and provide us with the resources to preserve the form of our bodies and blend into our busy life.

Body fat can be shed more easily than the agreed slow and steady method of 1-2 lb per week.

But commitment, involvement, and strict care for diet and a lot of high octane training are required. It also requires commitment and willingness to rest and recovery! What is really the limiting factor for many?

Apparently, overwork does not really occur–the term "under-recovery" should bere-specified. Rest, massages, vitamins, food, fluids and other athletes will practice hours of the day, but the majority of the day is always dedicated to rehabilitation.

The most important aspect in terms of fat loss is diet. Trained people are important, but eating takes longer and more knowledge, as all the work in a few moments can be lost very quickly. Train fast, eat better, don't lose fat than you need.

Train fairly hard, eat less and good: lose weight. The scheme of things makes it much easier to get enough exercise than to get the diet right-schedule three or four 45 minutes a week, have the equipment and a programme. Obviously, it's daunting to do so, but you just need to think about that 3 hours a week.

Nutrition, on the other hand, could be correct or incorrect in every moment! Many of us will always dream about hunger, or choose not to consume food, and this means that we are always starving and constantly fighting this famine!

Knowing how to relax our meals, how much we need to be mindful of our needs, and what we feel about our poor choices means that we can start taking care of this folly.

That makes the difference are our attitudes and tactics. The more weight you actually want to shed, the more likely you have to make lifestyle changes. The more you pick up the diet, the better your recovery, and the better you can bring your preparation into it.

But, for other people, you want to begin more slowly and over time build new habits. There can be an overwhelming notion of doing too much on one go and a turnaround, a sense of failure and self-interest. Baby steps will really produce amazing results.

The results are probably slower to launch, but studies show that the race is slow and steady in the long term.

If you are the type of person who has tried to make too many changes in one go, you can finally build life-long habit and behavior.

You're an important factor to consider. We have to play our strengths and don't always feel like someone else too much. If you're only inspired by major changes and a full rewrite, that's awesome! So long as the long-term view, the way you handle it shifts your mind.

When you notice too many changes too quickly, you are too early to figure out the roadmap and gradually build things.

It is important to note that **CONSISTENCE** still wins! Stalls or plateaus are more often than not related to traditions than to foods. We are self-sufficient and begin slack on stuff we were tight at the beginning. This is not a new plan we need–we will try to do what we have done better!

I'm just going to say, focus on FIRST patterns. Implement the fundamentals consistently and learn to balance tactics and good habits properly rather than to jump immediately to an ambitious strategy. After all, you may not have to do the most serious!

When you come to a point where you really want to improve items, or move them to a completely new level, the website offers more plans. Nonetheless, most people use the "serious" solutions first and see them as the magic bullet or quick fix. Many people try to use these methods unstoppably because the fundamentals are not dialed.

The basics might not seem exciting, but would you like to actually learn about intense diet and training for the rest of your life? Would you prefer simple routines and strategies that can be incorporated effortlessly into your life, which are almost easily praised for years to come? Think about it.

SUCCESS IS A SCIENCE;

IF YOU HAVE THE CONDITIONS,

YOU GET THE **RESULT**.

- Oscar Wilde -

...

THERE ARE NO SECRETS TO SUCCESS.

IT IS THE RESULT OF PREPARATION, HARD WORK,

AND LEARNING FROM FAILURE.

- Colin Powell -

CONCLUSION

Weight loss is not only a matter of diet and exercise, but the all-important but often overlooked psychological and emotional component. There has always been a link between diet and emotions that demonstrates how necessary it is to be inspired to lose weight.

Patterns, challenges, progress, defeat, setting goals for weight loss include, accomplishment of objectives, motivation and so on. Firstly-it begins and establishes an expectation or a goal.

Then there are preparations and tactics to carry out what you want. So perseverance follows, interacting confidently with you during times of disappointment and making arrangements for you, even when things look bad. That's the reason why you're inspired to lose weight; it's all about weight loss!

At some point, we have all heard the' mind over matter' claim that we seek to do anything, including losing weight, in life. But do we stop thinking what it really means? Are our mind so powerful that "matter" can be overcome? And if so, what is "matter" that we mean?

In most situations, "matter" for mind is anything that we have to resolve or gain, whether it is a lack of weight or a winning basketball match or something like that for the short term, when we have to go to the toilet very badly but have none to do.

"<u>Mind over Matter</u>" means that we can overcome any challenge or accomplish our objectives by using the energy of the mind to concentrate our attention on those objectives.

This means that if you use your mind's strength or "Mind over matter", working on your weight loss, fitness and nutritional objectives, it all allows you to stay on track and lose weight. So think about your habits, the benefits that weight loss will offer you and your body every day before your bed is even off and think about how easy it is to stick to your diet and exercise. As you eat, remind yourself how healthy your body is and how it will help you lose weight. Do this all day, and the influence of' mentality over matter' works for you, and you can watch pounds and centimeters go off easily.

I HOPE I HAVE HELPED YOU

WITH THIS SHORT GUIDE,

AND I WISH YOU A <u>WINNING LIFE</u>!

- Adam Clark -

See you on Amazon and don't miss my next book!